The Army Nurse Corps in World War

Judith A. Bellafaire

The Army Nurse Corps in World War

Table of Contents

The Army Nurse Corps in World War..**1**

    Judith A. Bellafaire..1

Introduction..1

The Army Nurse Corps in World War..2

    Early Operations in the Pacific..3

    Recruitment and Training..6

    Black Army Nurses..8

    At the Front..9

    The Chain of Evacuation...11

    Transport to General and Station Hospitals....................................12

    Sicily and Southern Italy..15

    Anzio..17

    The European Theater...19

    The Pacific Theater...23

    China–Burma–India Theater..28

    Conclusion...29

    Further Readings...31

The Army Nurse Corps in World War

Judith A. Bellafaire

Kessinger Publishing reprints thousands of hard–to–find books!

Visit us at http://www.kessinger.net

- The Army Nurse Corps in World War

    - Early Operations in the Pacific
    - Recruitment and Training
    - Black Army Nurses
    - At the Front
    - The Chain of Evacuation
    - Transport to General and Station Hospitals
    - Sicily and Southern Italy
    - Anzio
    - The European Theater
    - The Pacific Theater
    - China–Burma–India Theater
    - Conclusion

- Further Readings

Introduction

World War II was the largest and most violent armed conflict in the history of mankind. However, the half century that now separates us from that conflict has exacted its toll on our collective knowledge. While World War II continues to absorb the interest of military scholars and historians, as well as its veterans, a generation of Americans has grown to maturity largely unaware of the political, social, and military implications of a war that, more than any other, united us as a people with a common purpose.

Highly relevant today, World War II has much to teach us, not only about the profession of arms, but also about military preparedness, global strategy, and combined operations in the coalition war against fascism. During the next several years, the U.S. Army will participate in the nation's 50th anniversary commemoration of World War II. The commemoration will include the publication of various materials to help educate Americans about that war. The works produced will provide great opportunities to learn about and renew pride in an Army that fought so magnificently in what has been called "the mighty endeavor."

World War II was waged on land, on sea, and in the air over several diverse theaters of operation for approximately six years. The following essay on the critical support role of the Army Nurse Corps supplements a series of studies on the Army's campaigns of that war.

This brochure was prepared in the U.S. Army Center of Military History by Judith A. Bellafaire. I hope this absorbing account of that period will enhance your appreciation of American achievements during World War II.

GORDON R. SULLIVAN
General, United States Army
Chief of Staff

The Army Nurse Corps in World War

More than 59,000 American nurses served in the Army Nurse Corps during World War II. Nurses worked closer to the front lines than they ever had before. Within the "chain of evacuation" established by the Army Medical Department during the war, nurses served under fire in field hospitals and evacuation hospitals, on hospital trains and hospital ships, and as flight nurses on medical transport planes. The skill and dedication of these nurses contributed to the extremely low post–injury mortality rate among American military forces in every theater of the war. Overall, fewer than 4 percent of the American soldiers who received medical care in the field or underwent evacuation died from wounds or disease.

The tremendous manpower needs faced by the United States during World War II created numerous new social and economic opportunities for American women. Both society as a whole and the United States military found an increasing number of roles for women. As large numbers of women entered industry and many of the professions for the first time, the need for nurses clarified the status of the nursing profession. The Army reflected this changing attitude in June 1944 when it granted its nurses officers' commissions and full retirement privileges, dependents' allowances, and equal pay. Moreover, the government provided free education to nursing students between 1943 and 1948.

Military service took men and women from small towns and large cities across America and transported them around the world. Their wartime experiences broadened their lives as well as their expectations. After the war, many veterans, including nurses, took advantage of the increased educational opportunities provided for them by the government. World War II changed American society irrevocably and redefined the status and opportunities of the professional nurse.

Early Operations in the Pacific

The Army Nurse Corps listed fewer than 1,000 nurses on its rolls on 7 December 1941, the day of the Japanese surprise attack on Pearl Harbor. Eighty–two Army nurses were stationed in Hawaii serving at three Army medical facilities that infamous morning. Tripler Army Hospital was overwhelmed with hundreds of casualties suffering from severe burns and shock. The blood–spattered entrance stairs led to hallways where wounded men lay on the floor awaiting surgery. Army and Navy nurses and medics (enlisted men trained as orderlies) worked side by side with civilian nurses and doctors. As a steady stream of seriously wounded servicemen continued to arrive through the early afternoon, appalling shortages of medical supplies became apparent. Army doctrine kept medical supplies under lock and key, and bureaucratic delays prevented the immediate replacement of quickly used up stocks. Working under tremendous pressure, medical personnel faced shortages of instruments, suture material, and sterile supplies. Doctors performing major surgery passed scissors back and forth from one table to another. Doctors and nurses used cleaning rags as face masks and operated without gloves.

Nurses at Schofield Hospital and Hickam Field faced similar difficult circumstances. The chief nurse at Hickam Field, 1st Lt. Annie G. Fox, was the first of many Army nurses to receive the Purple Heart. Established by General George Washington during the Revolutionary War, this decoration originally was for "outstanding performance of duty and meritorious acts of extraordinary fidelity." After 1932, however, the medal was usually restricted to those wounded or injured by enemy action. Although unwounded, Lieutenant Fox received her medal for "her fine example of calmness, courage, and leadership, which was of great benefit to the morale of all she came in contact with." The citation foreshadowed the nurses' contribution to World War II.

Throughout 1941 the United States had responded to the increasing tensions in the Far East by deploying more troops in the Philippines. The number of Army nurses stationed on the islands grew proportionately to more than one hundred. Most nurses worked at Sternberg General Hospital in Manila and at Fort McKinley, 7 miles outside the city. However, a few nurses were at Fort Stotsenberg, 75 miles north of Manila, and two worked at Camp John Hay, located 200 miles to the north in the mountains. Several nurses worked on the island of Corregidor.

The Japanese attacked the Philippines on 8 December, Philippine time. Clark Field, adjacent to the Army hospital at Fort Stotsenberg, suffered a three-hour air raid during which planes, barracks, and field shops were bombed. The hospital escaped damage, but the large number of casualties from the air attack overwhelmed the small staff. The chief nurse at Sternberg sent several of her nurses to Stotsenberg to help cope with the emergency. They remained at Stotsenberg until 27 December when they received orders to evacuate to Manila. By that time Japanese forces had landed on the main island of Luzon and were approaching the city of Manila from the north. All of the nurses sta-

Page 5

tioned outside of Manila reached the city except for two nurses stranded at Camp John Hay, who were taken prisoner by the Japanese.

General Douglas MacArthur, commander of U.S. Army Forces in the Far East, declared Manila an open city and ordered the nurses to the island of Corregidor. MacArthur planned to hold Corregidor and the Bataan Peninsula and await supplies and reinforcement from the United States. He sent forty-five nurses from Corregidor to the Bataan Peninsula to prepare two emergency hospitals for U.S. and Filipino forces fighting on Bataan. General Hospital 1, near Limay, received casualties directly from the front lines. The hospital consisted of sixteen wooden buildings and was originally well supplied. More than 1,200 battle casualties requiring major surgery (traumatic amputations and head, chest, and abdominal wounds) were admitted to this hospital within a month.

Those patients strong enough for evacuation were sent to General Hospital 2, located near Cabcabin on the Real River. This hospital was out in the open, with no tents or buildings. Only a canopy of trees sheltered thousands of patients from Japanese aircraft.

The Japanese bombed Hospital 1 on 29 March, scoring a direct hit on the wards and killing or seriously wounding more than one hundred patients. A nurse remembered the force of the bomb. "The sergeant pulled me under the desk, but the desk was blown into the air, and he and I with it. I heard myself gasping. My eyes were being gouged out of their sockets, my whole body felt swollen and torn apart by the violent pressure. Then I fell back to the floor, and the desk landed on top of me and bounced around. The sergeant knocked it away from me, and gasping for breath, bruised and aching, sick from swallowing the smoke from the explosive, I dragged myself to my feet." The sight that met her eyes was appalling. Patients had been blown out of their beds. Bodies and severed limbs hung from the tree branches. Although the nurses knew that nothing could be done to prevent further air attacks, they carried on.

With each passing week the number of patients in both hospitals increased, and available supplies decreased. Lack of adequate food and clothing left American and Filipino troops susceptible to malaria, dysentery, beriberi, and dengue fever. Increasing numbers of troops suffered from malnutrition. By the end of March each hospital, built to accommodate 1,000 patients, was treating over 5,000.

The day before the U.S. and Filipino forces on Bataan surrendered to the Japanese, the Army evacuated its nurses to Malinta Tunnel Hospital on the island of Corregidor. Japanese pilots subjected the island to heavy bombing for weeks following the surrender of Bataan. One nurse recalled, "the air in the tunnels was thick with the smell of disinfectant and anesthetics, and there were too many people. Several times the power plant supplying the tunnel was hit, leaving us without electricity or lights. It was pretty ghastly in there, feeling the shock of each detonation, and never knowing when we would be in total darkness." Each shell or bomb which hit the area above the hospital loosened more dust and dirt and raised the dust level in the tunnel. Overcrowding further diminished air quality as the 500–bed hospital was expanded to 1,000 beds.

Once Maj. Gen. Jonathan M. Wainwright, commanding U.S. forces on Corregidor, decided that surrender was inevitable, he ordered as many nurses as possible evacuated to Australia. On 29 April twenty nurses left the island on two Navy planes. Only one of the planes reached Australia. The second made a forced landing on Mindanao Lake, and all aboard were taken prisoner by the Japanese. On 3 May a submarine picked up ten Army nurses, one Navy nurse, and the wife of a naval officer and took them to Australia. When the U.S. Army on Corregidor surrendered to the Japanese three days later, there were still fifty–five Army nurses working at Malinta Hospital.

In July the Japanese took the nurses to Santo Tomas Internment Camp in Manila where they joined the ten nurses whose plane had made a forced landing on Mindanao Lake. The sixty–seven nurses remained prisoners of war until U.S. troops liberated them in February 1945.

Recruitment and Training

Six months after the Japanese bombed Pearl Harbor, there were 12,000 nurses on duty in the Army Nurse Corps. Few of them had previous military experience, and the majority reported for duty ignorant of Army methods and protocol. Only in July 1943 did Lt. Gen. Brehon B. Somervell, Commanding General, Army Service Forces, authorize a formal four–week training course for all newly commissioned Army nurses. This program stressed Army organization; military customs and courtesies; field sanitation; defense against air, chemical, and mechanized attack; personnel administration; military requisitions and correspondence, and property responsibility. From July 1943 through September 1945 approximately 27,330 newly inducted nurses graduated from fifteen Army training centers.

Nurse anesthetists were in short supply in every theater of operations, so the Army developed a special training program for nurses

Page 7

U.S. Army nurse instructs Army medics on the proper method of giving an injection, Queensland, Australia, 1942. (DA photograph)

interested in that specialty. More than 2,000 nurses trained in a six–month course designed to teach them how to administer inhalation anesthesia, blood and blood derivatives, and oxygen therapy as well as how to recognize, prevent, and treat shock.

Nurses specializing in the care of psychiatric patients were also in great demand. One out of every twelve patients in Army hospitals was admitted for psychiatric care, and the Army discharged approximately 400,000 soldiers for psychiatric reasons. The Surgeon General developed a twelve–week program to train nurses in the care and medication of these patients.

Public health administrators as well as the American public believed that the increasing demands of the U.S. armed forces for nurses were responsible for a shortage of civilian nurses. Responding to these concerns in June 1943, Congress passed the Bolton Act, which set up the Cadet Nurse Corps program. The U.S. government subsidized the education of nursing students who promised that following graduation they would engage in essential military or civilian nursing for the duration of the war. The government also subsidized nursing schools willing to accelerate their program of study and provide student nurses with their primary training within two and a half years. Cadet nurses spent the last six months of their training assigned to civilian or military hospitals, which helped to alleviate the critical nursing shortage. Possible assignments included hospitals run by the Army, Navy, Veterans Administration, Public Health Service, and Bureau of Indian Affairs. The Cadet Nurse Corps training program was extremely successful and enjoyed enthusiastic public support. By 1948 when the program was discontinued, more than 150,000 nurse graduates testified to its value.

In December 1943 the U.S. War Department decided that there were enough nurses in the Army Nurse Corps to meet both existing and anticipated future demands on the Army. Consequently, the Army instructed the American Red Cross, which throughout the war had been responsible for the recruitment of nurses for the Army Nurse Corps, to stop recruiting. The Red Cross sent telegrams to local volunteer committees in every state advising them to discontinue their sustained drive to enlist nurses.

During the spring of 1944 intensive planning for the Allied invasion of France and the high number of anticipated casualties gave the Army second thoughts. Late in April the War Department advised the War Manpower Commission that it was revising its earlier decision to stop recruiting nurses. A new quota for the Army Nurse Corps was set at 50,000 10,000 more than were then enrolled. The Surgeon General promptly announced that the Army Nurse Corps was 10,000 nurses short, leading some critics to charge that American nurses were shirking their duty and avoiding military service. Yet nurses who responded to the much publicized "shortfall" and tried to enlist were hindered by the collapse of the local Red Cross recruiting networks.

In his January 1945 State of the Union Address President Franklin D. Roosevelt remarked that there was a critical shortage of Army nurses and that medical units in the European theater were being strained to the breaking point. He proposed that nurses be drafted. A nurse draft bill passed in the House and came within one vote in the Senate before the surrender of Germany. In the interim, the enrollment of over 10,000 nurses in the Army Nurse Corps early in 1945 rendered the measure superfluous.

Black Army Nurses

The Army Nurse Corps accepted only a small number of black nurses during World War II. When the war ended in September 1945 just 479 black nurses were serving in a corps of 50,000 because a quota system imposed by the segregated Army during the fast two years of the war held down the number of black enrollments. In 1943, for example, the Army limited the number of black nurses in the Nurse Corps to 160. Army authorities argued that assignments available to black nurses were limited because they were only allowed to care for black troops in black wards or hospitals. But unfavorable public reaction and political pressure forced the Army to drop its quota system in 1944. Subsequently, about 2,000 black students enrolled in the Cadet Nurse Corps program, and nursing schools for blacks benefited from increased federal funding.

The first black medical unit to deploy overseas was the 25th Station Hospital Unit, which contained thirty nurses. The unit went to Liberia in 1943 to care for U.S. troops protecting strategic airfields and rubber plantations. Malaria was the most serious health problem the troops encountered. Although malarial patients required an intensive amount of care, much of this work was routine and could be rendered by trained corpsmen. The nurses felt superfluous, and unit morale declined. The nurses were recalled late in 1943 because of poor health and low morale. Some were sent to general and station hospitals in the United States; others went to the 383d and 335th Station Hospitals near Tagap, Burma, where they treated black troops working on the Ledo Road. Another group of fifteen nurses deployed to the Southwest Pacific Area in the summer of 1943 with the all–black 268th Station Hospital. In June 1944 a unit of sixty–three nurses went to the 168th Station Hospital in England to care for German prisoners of war. By the end of the war, black nurses had served in Africa, England' Burma, and the Southwest Pacific.

At the Front

Early in the morning of 8 November 1942, sixty nurses attached to the 48th Surgical Hospital climbed over the side of a ship off the coast of North Africa and down an iron ladder into small assault boats. Each boat carried 5 nurses, 3 medical officers, and 20 enlisted men. The nurses wore helmets and carried full packs containing musette bags, gas masks, and canteen belts. Only their Red Cross arm bands and lack of weapons distinguished them from fighting troops. They waded ashore near the coastal town of Arzew on D–day of Operation TORCH with the rest of the assault troops and huddled behind a sand dune while enemy snipers took potshots at anything that moved. That evening they found shelter in some abandoned beach houses. These poorly constructed, noisome structures seemed like a safe haven in which to rest. Before the night was over, however, their commanding officer ordered them to an abandoned civilian hospital, where they began caring for invasion casualties. There was no electricity or running water, and the only medical supplies available were those the nurses had brought themselves. The hospital was under sporadic sniper fire. Doctors operated under flashlights held by nurses and enlisted men. There were not enough beds for all the casualties, and wounded soldiers lay on a concrete floor in pools of blood. Nurses dispensed what comfort they could, although the only sedatives available were the ones that they had carried with them during the landing because enemy air attacks on the harbor at Arzew delayed the unloading of supplies for two days.

The Army nurses who participated in the North African invasion at first had little conception of the realities of battle and were unfamiliar with military procedures. One nurse at the Arzew hospital became so incensed at snipers firing into the windows of the hospital and endangering the patients that she had to be forcibly restrained from going outside to "give them a piece of her mind." Several weeks later at the 48th Surgical Hospital in the hills near Tebessa, nurses sewed over fifty sheets into a large white cross to mark their installation as a hospital to enemy aircraft. The huge cross was on display only a short time when an Air Force officer told them that the cross, "the pride and joy of our hearts, which we were certain that the enemy would respect," identified the unit as an airfield under construction, making it a lucrative target. The nurses resumed sewing until they had made a large white square, in the center of which medical corpsmen painted a red cross, the proper identification. Episodes like these encouraged the Army to establish a training program for newly recruited nurses in 1943.

Nurses serving at the front in North Africa became expert at meeting the challenges of combat while caring for incoming patients. In February 1943 when news reached the 77th Evacuation Hospital bivouacked near Tebessa that the *German Army* had broken through the Kasserine Pass, staff members packed up and moved their 150 patients sixty miles to a safer bivouac. Within twelve hours a new hospital was fully operational and received another 500 casualties. During the Allied counterattack from mid–April through May 1943, which captured northern Tunisia, the 77th treated 4,577 soldiers within a 45–day period.

The head nurse of the 48th Surgical Hospital near Gaisa remembered that the hospital was situated between an ammunition dump and an airfield, both of which were primary targets for German bombers. The danger served to pull the doctors and nurses of the 48th Surgical together into a team based on mutual respect. Some Medical Corps doctors and corpsmen had believed that employing nurses so near the front lines would prove troublesome. Would nurses be able to perform their duties while under hostile fire? The work of the Army nurses, their dedication, and their professionalism more than proved their worth in the North African campaign, and they gained the respect of doctors, corpsmen, patients, and the military command.

The Chain of Evacuation

The Army Medical Department's newly organized and thus experimental "chain of evacuation" and the nurses' role in it were tested in North Africa and ultimately used successfully in every theater in the war. Critical were mobile field and evacuation hospitals, which closely followed the combat troops. These hospitals were usually set up in tents and were subject to move at short notice. Nurses packed and unpacked these hospitals each time they moved.

Litter bearers and ambulance drivers brought the wounded to field hospitals. Usually 18 nurses were assigned to a field hospital, which could handle 75 to 150 patients. Doctors and nurses performed triage on patients at the field hospital receiving tent. These evaluations were of critical importance. The severity of a patient's condition and the need for special treatment determined when, how, and where the patient was to be sent. Improper evacuation might result in the death of a patient from lack of immediate care. Those patients judged strong enough to travel were taken by ambulance to evacuation hospitals located farther away from the front lines and near transportation facilities. Nurses stabilized others with blood, plasma, medication, and dressings before sending them on. Patients who needed immediate care went directly into surgery. Those who needed surgery but were too weak for an immediate operation and could not travel were sent to the shock ward.

A field hospital could perform approximately eighty operations a day, and over 85 percent of those soldiers operated on in field hospitals survived. When postoperative patients grew strong enough, they were transported by ambulance to evacuation hospitals.

Evacuation hospitals had 53 nurses each and could accommodate up to 750 patients. Doctors operated on patients sent from field hospitals. Patients with postoperative stomach wounds were routinely kept in an evacuation hospital ten days before they were sent on, and those

 Page 13

with chest wounds were usually kept at least five days before they were evacuated. Critically wounded patients needing specialized treatment were air evacuated to station and general hospitals. Stable patients requiring a long recuperation were sent on via hospital ship.

Station and general hospitals advanced more slowly than field and evacuation hospitals and were usually housed in semipermanent locations. These hospitals were normally established in buildings with running water and electricity. Nurses sent to ready station and general hospitals in preparation for a new offensive often moved into abandoned, bombed-out hospitals, schools, or factories and became scrubwomen and scavengers in a hurried attempt to prepare for the expected inundation of battle casualties. Although personnel assigned to station and general hospitals did not experience enemy fire as often as those at the front, station and general hospitals were frequently subject to enemy air attacks.

Station hospitals received battle casualties from evacuation hospitals and performed surgery and specialized treatments. General hospitals were the last step in the evacuation line. Patients needing diagnosis, specialized lab tests, or long periods of recuperation and therapy were sent to general hospitals. Upon release patients were reclassified and either returned to duty or sent back to the United States. Both station and general hospitals also accepted patients from outside the chain of evacuation, such as servicemen and women who needed treatment for pneumonia or various contagious diseases.

Transport to General and Station Hospitals

Patients were evacuated from the field to station and general hospitals in the zone of communications via hospital trains, hospital ships, and aircraft. Nurses served on all these modes of transportation. On hospital trains they dispensed medication and food and made their patients as comfortable as possible, while watching them carefully for signs of stress and complications. Such trains usually had thirty-two beds per car, with one nurse assigned to each car of litter patients or to several cars of ambulatory patients.

Hospital ships operated under the terms of the Hague Convention which meant that those vessels could carry only military personnel on patient status accompanied by attending Medical and Transportation Corps personnel. The white hospital ships with large red crosses painted on either side were forbidden to carry cargo of any kind and were subject to enemy inspection at any time. Nevertheless, the Axis Powers

Flight nurse attends a wounded soldier being evacuated by air from the 57th Field Hospital in Prestwick, Scotland, 1944. (DA photograph)

did not always spare hospital ships, which were bombed in at least three different incidents. Army nurses were wounded when the Germans bombed hospital ships during the Allied invasions of Italy and Anzio. In the Pacific, Japanese pilots attacked the USS *Comfort* off Leyte Island in April 1945, seriously damaging the ship and killing twenty–nine people, including six Army nurses.

Air evacuation of patients began in North Africa in February 1943 and eventually became a feature of every theater of war. Flight nurses received special training before assignment to the Air Forces Surgeon General's Office. Training emphasized crash procedures, field survival in ocean, jungle, desert, and arctic environments, and the effects of high altitude on various types of patients. The rigors of patient care during flights demanded these nurses be in peak physical condition. Flight nurses assumed greater risks than their counterparts because the C–46, C–47, and C–54 transport planes used in patient evacuations doubled as cargo planes. For this reason they could not display the markings of the Geneva Red Cross to protect them from enemy fire. Besides the hazards of enemy fire, operational realities created difficulties for flight nurses. Pilots nicknamed the C–46 the "flying coffin" because heater problems sometimes caused these coffin–shaped planes to explode during flight. Some pilots refused to turn on the heaters in these planes, even when they were carrying patients. This complicated nursing care because critically ill patients cannot tolerate low temperatures. Nurses improvised and kept their patients warm with blankets and hot drinks.

An evacuation plane could be loaded and airborne within ten minutes. Usually one nurse and one medical corpsman were assigned to a flight. A doctor briefed the nurse on each patient's condition prior to takeoff, and during the flight she was responsible for the safety and comfort of up to twenty–five patients.

While in flight the nurse watched for anxiety attacks because many soldiers had never flown before. She checked each patient's pulse, respiration, and bleeding and adjusted and applied bandages and dressings, relieved pain, administered oxygen, and cared for those who became airsick. A bout of airsickness could be fatal to a patient with a broken jaw that had been wired shut. Nurses often gave such patients enough medication to encourage sleep throughout the trip. Some soldiers suffering from "battle fatigue" were so emotionally disturbed that they had to travel under restraint. Nurses could handle only a few of these "locked litter" patients per flight.

Frequent snarls in communication sometimes caused nurses to fly into an area aboard a plane loaded with ammunition only to discover that there were no patients waiting to be evacuated. On the return trip, the empty plane and its crew remained vulnerable to an enemy attack. Equally frustrating was the lack of emergency equipment on many evacuation aircraft. One nurse was faced with a patient who started bleeding beneath his plaster cast. There were no cast cutters on the plane, so the nurse had to hack away at the cast with bandage scissors, all the while watching the red stain spread ominously. She eventually removed the cast, stopped the bleeding, and stabilized the patient.

Flight nurses accepted that there would always be unexpected dangers. A transport plane en route to Guadalcanal with twenty–four litter patients and one flight nurse ran out of fuel over the Pacific. The pilot spotted an island on which there was a 150–foot–square clearing ringed with coconut palms and decided to crash land there rather than risk plunging into the ocean. During the landing, one passenger's windpipe was severed, although his jugular vein remained intact. The attending nurse quickly devised a suction tube from a syringe, a colonic tube, and the inflation tubes from a life jacket. With these tools, she was able to keep the man's windpipe clear of blood until help arrived nineteen hours later.

It is a tribute to the 500 Army nurses who served as members of 31 medical air evacuation transport squadrons operating worldwide that only 46 of the 1,176,048 patients air evacuated throughout the war died en route. Rapid evacuation by plane did lower the battle casualty fatality rate, but it cost the lives of 17 flight nurses during the war.

Sicily and Southern Italy

The nurses' performance during the North African invasion taught the Army several lessons that it applied to the invasions of Sicily and southern Italy. Commanding officers noticed that nurses acclimated quickly to difficult and dangerous conditions with a minimum of complaints. Their efficiency and professional accomplishments made them essential members of the field armies. The presence of nurses at the front improved the morale of all fighting men because soldiers realized that they would receive skilled care in the event they were wounded. Hospitalized men recovered sooner when nurses cared for them. Troops in the field figured that "if the nurses can take it, then we can."

U.S. and British troops invaded Sicily on 9 July 1943, and nurses of the 10th Field Hospital and the 11th Evacuation Hospital arrived on the island three days later. There they were greeted by German Stuka dive bombers which forced them into slit trenches and foxholes during the first few days. Other nurses scheduled to support the invading U.S. Seventh Army had to wait nine days for transport, which was in short supply during the first week of the invasion.

The intense heat on Sicily affected everyone, and the 128th Evacuation Hospital established at Cefalu (east of Palermo) saw increasing numbers of soldiers with malaria. Nurses lined the tents with mosquito netting in an attempt to control the spread of the disease through the hospital, but eventually medical personnel also succumbed. Despite the malaria epidemic, nurses at this hospital worked twelve–hour shifts. Teams of specialists (doctors and nurses) handled a spectrum of wounds including head, chest, and orthopedic as well as shock cases. Patient turnover was high. The hospital would admit 300 patients in one 24–hour period and evacuate 200 to North Africa for further treatment. Most patients went by train to the coast where they were placed on hospital ships. Critically ill patients were evacuated by plane.

The Army Nurse Corps in World War

Lt. Gen. Mark W. Clark originally planned that nurses should land with the troops during the 8 September invasion of the Italian mainland and care for the men as they had done in North Africa. However, after the Allies decided to land at Salerno rather than Reggio, General Dwight D. Eisenhower, Commander in Chief, Allied Expeditionary Force, decided to postpone the nurses' arrival. The Salerno beachhead was small, and there were few exits off the beaches. Eisenhower and his advisers believed that the beachhead would be heavily defended and that the nurses should wait until the landing force was secure.

On the night of 13 September German planes bombed the British hospital ship H.M.S. *Newfoundland* while it was en route to Salerno carrying the nurses. Bands of green lights and brilliantly illuminated red crosses clearly identified the *Newfoundland* as a hospital ship. Before the ship sank, British vessels rescued all 103 nurses aboard and evacuated them to Bizerte, Tunisia. Four nurses suffered minor wounds for which the Army later awarded them the Purple Heart. The others boarded another ship and arrived at Salerno ten days later.

The winter rains, which usually arrive in southern Italy in November, came one month early in 1943, making it very difficult to maintain adequate medical facilities under canvas. Three days after the nurses arrived at Salerno a severe storm knocked down the tents of the 16th Evacuation Hospital, housing approximately 1,000 patients. Nurses evacuated the drenched patients to an abandoned tobacco warehouse without incident, preventing complications from exposure.

Continuous bad weather caused one of the most famous incidents in Nurse Corps history. On 8 November 1943, a C–54 ferrying thirteen flight nurses and thirteen medical technicians (corpsmen) of the 807th Medical Air Evacuation Transport Squadron from Sicily to Bari on the east coast of Italy ran into severe weather. The plane lost radio contact, the compass failed, and the pilot became disoriented in the storm. Icing finally forced the plane down in the Albanian mountains far behind German lines. Partisan guerrillas found the Americans and took them to a nearby farmhouse. That night the flight crew set fire to the plane to conceal traces of their presence in the area.

The partisans escorted the fugitives through the mountains on foot to safety behind Allied lines. In bitterly cold weather and blinding snowstorms, the small band made a hazardous, two–month journey covering 800 miles. The escapees suffered from frostbite, dysentery, jaundice, and pneumonia, but all the nurses except three who were separated from the main body of the group arrived safely at Bari on 9 January.

The three missing nurses faced different hardships. A German unit trapped them for several months in the partisan town of Berat in the home of a partisan guerrilla. Dressed as Albanian civilians and supplied with Albanian identification cards, the nurses finally left Berat by car in March. They traveled far into the countryside, where partisans gave them donkeys to ride and escorted them across several mountain ranges. When they reached the coast, an Allied torpedo boat took them to Otranto, Italy. With their arrival at Otranto on 21 March, the three nurses completed a five–month sojourn behind enemy lines. The courage and fortitude of the "Balkan Nurses" on their 800–mile hike behind enemy lines provided an example of the Army nurse's ability to withstand hardships "at the front."

Anzio

To speed up the slow pace of the Allied northward advance through Italy against the fierce German defenses at Cassino and the Gustav Line, Allied strategists planned a landing behind the German lines. On 22 January the British and American troops launched a successful surprise attack and landing on the Anzio beachhead. Because surprise was complete, the projected 12 percent casualty rate was held to less than 1 percent throughout the initial landing. The Germans, however, quickly regrouped for a stubborn defense that pinned the Allied forces in the beachhead for four months and stalled hopes for a rapid advance. Within the congested invasion perimeter, casualties mounted as the Allies repulsed persistent *Luftwaffe* and ground attacks.

The 33d Field Hospital and the 95th and 96th Evacuation Hospitals landed with the Anzio beachhead assault force and quickly set up operations. Approximately two hundred nurses were assigned to these units. On 24 January 1944, two days after the landing, the first bombs fell near the medical facilities. That night three British hospital ships, H.M.S. *St. David,* H.M.S. *St. Andrew,* and H.M.S. *Leinster,* were attacked by *Luftwaffe* aircraft while evacuating casualties from the beachhead. As in the case of the *Newfoundland,* the ships were well lighted and clearly marked with the red cross. The *St. David,* with 226 medical staff and patients aboard, received a direct hit and sank. The two Army nurses on board were among 130 survivors rescued by the damaged *Leinster.* One of these nurses, 2d Lt. Ruth Hindman, had survived the earlier bombing of the *Newfoundland.*

The Army Nurse Corps in World War

On 7 February a German plane attempting to bomb the port at Anzio was intercepted by a British Spitfire. While trying to gain altitude, the German pilot jettisoned his antipersonnel bombs on the 95th Evacuation Hospital. The direct hit on the surgical section killed 26 staff and patients, including 3 nurses; 64 others were wounded. The day before, several news correspondents had decided among themselves that the constant shelling had rendered one nurse too nervous to carry on much longer. Yet after the bombing, this nurse calmly took charge, rallied the surviving staff (nurses and corpsmen), and guided their treatment of the wounded. Nevertheless the commander of the medical installations in the Mediterranean theater decided that the 95th Evacuation Hospital had lost too many key personnel to function effectively. He replaced the unit with the 15th Evacuation Hospital, formerly stationed at Cassino. The 15th arrived at Anzio on 10 February, just in time to witness the bombing of the 33d Field Hospital. Long–range enemy artillery fire killed 2 nurses and I enlisted man and wounded 4 medical officers and 7 enlisted men. Both nurses were off duty at the time of the attack. One nurse had stopped at the tent of the other to borrow a book when a shell hit the tent, killing them instantly. Meanwhile, another shell smashed the generator of the operating tent, which caught fire. Medical personnel evacuated the forty–two patients by flashlight without incident, and for their bravery four nurses–1st Lt. Mary Roberts, 2d Lt. Elaine Roe, 2d Lt. Virginia Rourke, and 2d Lt. Ellen Ainsworth– received the first Silver Star medals awarded to women in the U.S. Army. Ainsworth, who was killed during the attack, was awarded the medal posthumously.

Throughout February and March, medical installations on the beachhead continued to receive direct hits. On 29 March the 56th Evacuation Hospital was shelled, leaving 3 officers, 1 nurse, 14 enlisted men, and 19 patients wounded and 4 patients killed. Whenever the air raid sirens at Anzio sounded, those patients who could put on their steel helmets and crawled under their cots to avoid flying shrapnel. Nurses and corpsmen lifted others to the ground. Patients whose condition rendered them immovable became very nervous, and nurses ignored the danger to stay with them.

In April the 36th Engineer Regiment excavated 3 1/2–foot foundations for the hospital tents and reinforced these protective earthworks with sandbag walls. Patients and medical personnel inside the hospitals were finally protected from flying shrapnel although not from direct hits.

A later observer explained that the medical detachment at Anzio was "part of a front that had no back. The beachhead was 15 miles wide and 7 miles deep and allowed no retreat from enemy fire." The large, impassable Pontine Marsh forced the invaders to locate their antiaircraft batteries, airstrips, maintenance shops, food' gasoline, and ammunition dumps (all lucrative targets) on the edge of the medical area. Enemy bombers often missed their targets and hit the hospitals. The frequent enemy hits on the congested corner occupied by the main medical installations earned it the nickname "Hell's Half Acre." Many soldiers believed that they were safer in their frontline foxholes than they would be in the hospitals.

The Fifth Army command allowed the nurses to remain at Anzio regardless of the danger and the mounting casualties because they were desperately needed. Between January and June the Anzio field and evacuation hospitals admitted 25,809 battle casualties, 4,245 accidental injuries, and 18,074 medical casualties (disease). These soldiers were stabilized and evacuated rapidly and efficiently. The performance of Army nurses at Anzio reinforced the fact that women could function effectively under fire on the front lines.

The European Theater

By June 1945 the number of Army nurses in the European theater of the war reached a peak of 17,345. The first nurses to arrive in Normandy were members of the 42d and 45th Field Hospitals and the 91st and 128th Evacuation Hospitals. They landed on the beachhead four days after the initial invasion in June 1944.

The nurses' experiences in the European theater varied widely, depending upon their assignments. The experiences of those assigned to the 12th Evacuation Hospital reflected that diversity. Unit members sailed for England in January 1943. After several moves they arrived on the east coast of England in May 1944. There they participated in the buildup for the Allied invasion of the Continent by establishing a tent hospital and preparing for the expected influx of casualties. In early June they watched hundreds of Allied planes fly overhead to prepare the way for the invasion of the Continent on 6 June 1944. The first battle casualties arrived at the 12th Evacuation Hospital the next day, including members of the 101st Airborne Division and the 90th Infantry Division. The hospital admitted 1,309 patients and conducted 596 surgical operations before it displaced across the Channel.

The 12th Evacuation Hospital deployed to France in July, arriving in Normandy on I August. By that time most of the heavy casualties incurred during the first weeks of the invasion had already been evacuated to England. Throughout August Allied forces pushed the *German Briny* eastward through France toward the Siegfried Line. The front moved rapidly; high numbers of casualties occurred only in pockets of resistance and were handled by other evacuation hospitals. The 12th found that it was not needed. Nonetheless, for almost a month the 12th Evacuation Hospital followed the troops through France. Transportation facilities were strained to the limit, and the unit encountered frequent delays. This was a frustrating time for the nurses. They often slept out in the open without tents, spent days looking for their equipment, and suffered from boredom and inactivity.

In mid–September the Allies met the German defenses at the Siegfried Line, and casualties mounted. The 12th established operations at Bonneval, where it admitted 1,260 patients in less than one month. It then received orders to deploy to Rheims and operate in the abandoned American Memorial Hospital, which the retreating Germans had left in poor condition. After the nurses spent several days scrubbing and cleaning, they received orders to turn over the American Memorial to another medical unit and to establish an evacuation hospital in a field near the Argonne Forest. They remained there for a month, then moving into a hospital building in the town of Nancy where the unit wintered. Although the Germans shelled the town regularly, the hospital suffered but a single hit and that shell failed to explode. In early 1945 the unit was again on the move to Luxembourg.

The nurses of the 12th moved eleven times in two years. After each relocation they had to prepare a sanitary, comfortable hospital capable of handling large numbers of critically wounded or sick patients. Their experience alternated between periods of exhausting activity and intense boredom. They had to be flexible, innovative, quick–thinking, patient, adaptable, and highly skilled. Their experi–

Page 22

ences were similar to those of nurses in field and evacuation hospitals everywhere in Europe.

The Army Nurse Corps in World War

Nurses frequently demonstrated their ability to remain calm in unpredictable and dangerous situations. For example, flight nurse Reba Z. Whittle's C–47 was caught by flak and crashed behind enemy lines in September 1944. Every member of the crew, including Whittle, was wounded. The Germans provided their prisoners with medical care and upon their recovery incarcerated them in Stalag IXC. Whittle's captors allowed her to nurse other POWs throughout her captivity. Whittle was held as a prisoner of war for five months until her release in January 1945.

Although the chain of evacuation necessitated frequent patient turnover, nurses in the field provided long–term, intensive care when necessary. For example, from September through December 1944 the 77th Evacuation Hospital received numerous casualties from troops attempting to clear the Germans from the Huertgen Forest. Four U.S. infantry divisions were sent into the rugged woods, and each suffered appalling casualties. The area consisted of steep hills covered in thick evergreens and hedged about by barbed wire and mines. Men arrived at the hospital suffering from trench foot, exhaustion, and exposure. By December trench foot accounted for more casualties than all other causes combined. The disease manifested itself when troops were confined in foxholes for over forty–eight hours, their feet cold, wet, and immobile. Casualties arrived at the hospital unable to walk. The condition was extremely painful and demanded a high level of nursing care.

In December 1944 the *German Army* under Field Marshal General Gerd von Rundstedt launched an all–out offensive against the western front, popularly known as the Battle of the Bulge. The German attack bowed the American front line westward almost to the Meuse River. Many medical units, among them the 44th and the 67th Evacuation Hospitals, were forced to evacuate the area on short notice. Five nurses with the 67th volunteered to stay overnight with 200 patients too weak to withstand the move. All night they listened to the approaching roar of the German guns as they cared for their patients. The next day the Army evacuated nurses and patients within hours of the Germans' arrival.

German aircraft struck several medical installations in the course of the offensive. On 17 December bombs hit the 76th General Hospital, located in the town of Liege. The 77th Evacuation Hospital Unit had set up operations in a school building in the nearby town of Verviers, an important transportation junction just north of the Bulge. When the Germans bombed Verviers on the night of 20 December, the south corner of the hospital building was hit. The nurses' quarters, laboratory, and pharmacy all sustained severe damage. Fortunately, only one nurse was injured in the attack.

After American and British forces repulsed this last German offensive, medical units accompanied the Allied forces into Germany. In newly conquered, hostile territory the nurses experienced new pressures. Third Army nurses noticed that the deeper the Americans went into Germany, the more openly hostile German civilians became. Near Darmstadt, the hospital had to be guarded at all times. According to one nurse, German civilians looked at the nurses "with actual hatred in their eyes–and children throw stones at ambulances and spit at jeeps."

On Easter Sunday 1945, near the town of Hanau, a hospital convoy, its lead jeep plainly marked with a white flag bearing the Geneva Cross, was ambushed by a company of the *German 6th SS Mountain Division.* The *SS* troops burst out of the forest firing machine guns. Medical personnel, including ten nurses, took cover in the nearest ditch. All came out with their hands over their heads when ordered, and the Germans marched them into the woods. The Germans confiscated the unit's vehicles and all the hospital equipment and took their prisoners to a nearby nursing home, where they ordered them to set up a hospital for German wounded. The Americans did the best they could without any of their equipment, and the nurses worked calmly under enemy guns. Nine hours later troops of the U.S. 5th Infantry Division liberated all the prisoners from their short but harrowing period of captivity.

The final push into central Germany cost the western Allies heavy casualties and required medical units to work under great pressure. The 44th Evacuation Hospital admitted 1,348 patients from the 3d Armored Division during one 56–hour period in mid–April. Casualties also came in from the 9th Infantry, engaged in clearing out the area north of the Harz Mountains.

When American and British paratroopers who had been prisoners of the Germans were rescued, the 77th Evacuation Hospital received them. Most were weak and malnourished, and the medical care they had received while in captivity was inferior by American standards. Nurses had to remove casts and dressings and apply newer, more comfortable ones. A different problem was presented by the increasing numbers of German POWs. At first, some nurses wondered if they were capable of putting personal feelings aside and providing these patients with the best care available. Moreover, offi– cial theater hospital policy clearly placed the care of Allied casualties over that offered to enemy prisoners. Most nurses, however, quickly discovered that they were able to view these men simply as patients in need of care and treated Germans no differently than American soldiers. Nurses screened enemy casualties away from Allied patients to make all more comfortable.

Army nurses of the 116th and 127th Evacuation Hospitals cared for concentration camp victims liberated from Dachau. These patients needed special care and constant attention and reassurance. Many clung to nurses as their saviors and would not let them out of their sight. Victims of starvation, with long–neglected wounds inflicted by systematic torture, many also suffered from typhus, frozen feet, gangrene, bed sores, and severe dermatitis. Eight out of every ten inmates had tuberculosis. Despite intensive care, many died from weakness, malnutrition, and disease.

The Pacific Theater

Army nurses worked near the front lines under fire in the European and Mediterranean theaters. Their courage under the most adverse conditions at Anzio, uncomplaining resilience in the Balkans, and calm professionalism in Germany demonstrated that they should be considered essential elements of the U.S. Army in any theater of operations. Nevertheless, Pacific theater commanders limited the Army nurses' combat support role to rear areas because they did not feel comfortable assigning American women to uncivilized jungle areas where they would be vulnerable to Japanese guerrilla attacks. The decision, unpopular from beginning to end, understandably resulted in morale problems for both nurses and soldiers.

Army nurses served throughout the Pacific in increasing numbers between 7 December 1941 and the end of the war. Nurses usually found themselves assigned to hospitals far from combat areas where they cared for soldiers who had been evacuated from the front lines. Due to the island–hopping nature of the Pacific campaign, Army nurses were stationed in the Hawaiian Islands, Australia, New Zealand, the Fiji Islands, New Caledonia, and the New Hebrides in 1942 but did not arrive in combat areas until after the fighting ceased. They followed one step behind the U.S. troops, arriving on an island only after it had fallen under Allied control. Nurses were stationed in areas that were outside a direct Japanese ground threat, yet near enough to the front lines to receive air evacuees. New Caledonia became home to seven station and two general hospitals because the climate was mild and the island was malaria free. More nurses served on New Caledonia and remained there longer than on any other Pacific island except for Australia and Hawaii. The first nurses to see the island were those of the 9th and 109th Station Hospitals and the 52d Evacuation Hospital, who arrived in New Caledonia in March 1942. Both the hospitals and the nurses' quarters were prefabricated buildings with electricity and running water. Some nurses complained about the six–inch–deep mud and torrential downpours, but many eventually became bored with their relatively placid assignment and longed to serve closer to the troops where there was more excitement.

The hospitals on New Caledonia received malaria cases from Guadalcanal, the Solomon Islands, and the New Hebrides. More than 50 percent of admissions for disease between 1942 and 1944 were malaria patients. Battle casualties arriving from New Guinea, New Britain, Guadalcanal, and Saipan were predominantly abdominal cases, but chest wounds were also common.

Like the nurses working on New Caledonia, those stationed on New Zealand, the Fiji Islands, and the New Hebrides between 1942 and 1944 also received casualties evacuated from the front lines via plane and hospital ship. Malaria was endemic to the New Hebrides, and both nurses and patients were susceptible to this debilitating disease. The hospitals in New Zealand, Fiji, and the New Hebrides closed down in 1944, and the nurses moved on to the Solomon Islands, the Marshall Islands, and the Marianas, arriving only after Allied forces had gained control. Once again, they cared for soldiers who had been air evacuated from frontline areas.

Medical corpsmen who had served in place of nurses in combat zones sometimes resented the nurses' arrival. "Once the nurses arrive, the morale of the corpsmen plummets," said one observer. The nurses took over skilled direct–care tasks and relegated the corpsmen to lesser duties and scrub work. Nurses commanded corpsmen in the chain of command because the nurses were trained professionals while corpsmen usually had only minimal training. Friction between nurses and corpsmen had been absent in the North African and European theaters, where nurses followed combat troops much more closely. In the Pacific, however, commanders appeared more concerned with sheltering the nurses from the vicissitudes of war and proved unwilling to take responsibility for placing them anywhere near the combat zone.

The Army Nurse Corps in World War

Nurses stationed on the secured islands of Guadalcanal, New Guinea, Saipan, Guam, and Tinian found their quarters fenced in and guarded by armed guards twenty–four hours a day. They were escorted to and from the hospital and could not leave their quarters during their free time unless they were part of a supervised group activity. The island commands enforced evening curfews and required nurses to have an armed escort after 1800 (6:00 P.M.).Two armed guards accompanied any nurse who traveled off post.

Women's Army Corps (WAC) members stationed on these islands received the same treatment. American women represented a tiny minority of the personnel in these areas, and General MacArthur wanted to protect the women for whom he had responsibility. The official policy was that the women were guarded because isolated Japanese guerrilla patrols still roamed the islands. In reality, however, Army leadership hoped to discourage incidents of sexual harassment and fraternization.

The first nurses to arrive on New Guinea were those of the 153d Station Hospital, who reached Port Moresby in October 1942. The 10th Evacuation Hospital and the 171st Station Hospital reached the island in December. These hospitals cared for casualties from the Buna–Gona campaign from November 1942 through January 1943.

Nurses of the 20th Station Hospital arrived on Guadalcanal in June 1944. Male medical personnel of the unit had been on the island since January 1943. The nurses of the 20th were soon followed by those of the 48th Station Hospital, the 9th Station Hospital, and the 137th Station Hospital.

Both Guadalcanal and New Guinea were hot, humid, rainy, and extremely uncomfortable. The tropical climate encouraged malaria, scrub typhus, dengue fever, and tropical dysentery, which together caused four times as many casualties as did battle wounds. The nurses also encountered yaws, leprosy, bubonic plague, and cutaneous diphtheria, diseases with which they had had little if any experience.

By January 1943 there were 14,646 American troops on New Guinea, 8,659 of whom had contracted some form of disease, with malaria being the most common. Army leaders instituted strict malarial control methods on New Guinea, Guadalcanal, and the New Hebrides. Personnel were required to wear protective clothing after sundown. Buildings were screened, and medical malarial control units sprayed DDT across the islands. By 1945 the theater–wide malarial rate was lowered from 172 per thousand to under 5 per thousand.

Air raid alerts were commonplace on New Guinea but actual bombings rare. On 24 November 1943, a Japanese plane dropped four incendiary and four high–explosive bombs on the 153d Station Hospital area. Two hospital tents were damaged and two were knocked down, but only three minor casualties resulted among personnel. On 8 December the 153d was again strafed and bombed by twenty Japanese planes supposedly celebrating the anniversary of Pearl Harbor. Once more there were only a few minor injuries and no casualties.

Nurses arrived on Saipan, an island in the Marianas chain, in July 1944, only one month after the Americans invaded the island. The first nurses on Saipan were attached to the 369th Station Hospital. Nurses of the 148th General Hospital and the 176th Station Hospital joined them in August. Throughout 1944 the nurses saw a pattern similar to that experienced by nurses on New Guinea and Guadalcanal, with five admissions for disease to every battle casualty. An epidemic of dengue fever hit the medical installations in Saipan during the late summer of 1944, and half the nurses on the island suffered from the disease. The epidemic was controlled only after the Army sprayed DDT across the entire island in September. Although Japanese planes bombed and strafed the island of Saipan in late 1944, there were no American casualties. In early 1945 and throughout the fighting on Iwo Jima and Okinawa, the hospitals on Saipan suffered from a severe water shortage. Water had to be rationed and hand carried to wards from outside drums.

On 4 December 1944, nurses of the 289th Station Hospital disembarked on the island of Guam in the Marianas. Three days later they were followed by sixty–three nurses of the 373d Station Hospital. Finally on 28 December the personnel of the 204th General Hospital arrived on the island.

The 374th Station Hospital was established on the island of Tinian in the Marianas in late January 1945. One month after the arrival of the 374th, the hospitals on Saipan, Guam, and Tinian began receiving battle casualties from Iwo Jima. Over 18,000 casualties arrived within a single month. After Iwo Jima was secured in late March, the Okinawa campaign began almost immediately. For the Allies, the island of Okinawa was the last step toward the main islands of Japan. But Okinawa was fiercely defended. Within three months, from April to June 1945, more than 50,000 U.S. soldiers, sailors, and marines were wounded and 15,000 killed. Casualties sustained during the Okinawa campaign were evacuated to Guam, Saipan, and Tinian via plane and hospital ship. Although the twenty–four flight nurses stationed at Guam went on 273 missions during which they cared for 5,529 sick and wounded patients from the front lines to Guam, Saipan, or Tinian, the vast majority of Okinawa casualties arrived at the station and general hospitals of the Mariana Islands by hospital ship.

Nurses stationed on the Marianas worked twelve–hour days, seven days a week. Many patients arrived in severe shock, others in hemorrhage. Some had sustained multiple wounds, and many required traumatic amputations. Nurses assumed responsibilities handled by doctors in the United States. They gave transfusions, debrided and dressed wounds, and removed sutures. Nurses trained wardmen to give infusions and change dressings, duties traditionally reserved for nursing personnel.

Medical personnel set up special wards for the many severely burned patients who had been on oil tankers attacked by Japanese suicide planes. Nurses stabilized burn patients with plasma, blood, and morphine in the shock ward before taking them into surgery for debridement and Vaseline pressure dressings.

As the Okinawa campaign drew to a close, the 232d General Hospital, including eighty–one nurses, was established on the island of Iwo Jima. The Japanese bombed and strafed the hospital periodically. Nurses who were off duty took refuge in two air raid shelters located in back of the nurses' quarters. Those who were on duty stayed with the patients and settled them in a cave located behind the hospital.

The invasion of the Philippines was the first opportunity for Army nurses in the Pacific theater to care for battle casualties in the field rather than patients evacuated from the front lines. With this change of policy, morale among the nurses improved substantially, and many nurses refused offers of rotation back to the United States. Army nurses arrived on Leyte Island with the 1st and 2d Field Hospitals nine days after the initial invasion on 20 October 1944. Within three hours after landing, they were administering medical care to the wounded in a former Catholic cathedral in Tacloban. Medical personnel on Leyte saw the highest ratio of killed to wounded casualties in the war, a tragic 1:3. Between January and February 1945, 19,257 patients were admitted to the hospitals on Leyte. Nurses treated many casualties from the kamikaze attacks on Liberty ships attempting to enter the harbor at Leyte. Between October and December 1944, almost 3,000 such casualties were evacuated from Leyte to New Guinea.

On 28 April 1945, a Japanese suicide plane bombed the hospital ship USS *Comfort* off Leyte Island. In the attack 6 nurses, 5 medical officers, 8 enlisted men, and 7 patients were killed, and 4 nurses were wounded. The ship was severely damaged but managed to enter the harbor at Guam under destroyer escort.

The Army nurse in the Pacific theater performed her tasks efficiently, compassionately, and courageously whether she was caring for casualties in the field or patients evacuated from the front lines. These nurses prevailed over dangers and difficulties not experienced by nurses in other theaters. They became ill with malaria and dengue fever; experienced the rigors of a tropical climate; tolerated water shortages; risked kamikaze attacks; adapted to curfews, fenced compounds, and armed escorts; and dealt with medical corpsmen's hostility. Nurses in the Pacific demonstrated their ability to overcome adversity and reached the front lines of a uniquely dangerous theater before the end of the war.

China–Burma–India Theater

A small number of Army nurses were stationed in Army hospitals in China, Burma, and India throughout 1943 and 1944, where they treated the American and Chinese troops who were pushing into southern China along the Ledo Road. At the time, the road was the sole overland lifeline for military supplies to Chiang Kai–shek's Chinese Nationalist Army, which was fighting a war of survival against Japan.

American nurses and Chinese patients experienced a clash of cultures which made the nurses' jobs difficult. The Chinese patients had difficulty understanding the concept of a "high–type" woman performing "menial" bedside care. The nurses found it hard to maintain proper discipline among the wards because the Chinese did not feel it necessary to follow a woman's orders. A nurse assigned to the 20th General Hospital remembered that her Chinese patients insisted on supplying their own food while in the hospital. The result was "orange peels, egg shells, chicken feathers, and vegetable peelings piled high beside each bed." Nurses could not keep their seriously sick patients in bed. "They wandered off to the bazaar in their pajamas to haggle over fresh vegetables, and live ducks and chickens, which they brought back to the wards and kept under their beds." Many patients refused to consume their atabrine tablets and contracted malaria. The most serious problem the nurses had, however, was that Chinese patients with contagious diseases refused to remain isolated from their fellows and thus inadvertently spread diseases throughout the hospital.

For every Allied soldier wounded in the struggle for Burma in 1943, 120 fell sick. The malarial rate that year was a staggering 84 percent of total manpower. The Army sprayed DDT on mosquito–infested areas and ordered all personnel to wear protective clothing after dusk regardless of the temperature. Troops were issued daily medication to protect them against malaria. Scrub typhus, a disease spread by mites, posed another problem. This disease demanded an extremely high level of nursing care and had a 30 percent fatality rate.

Although the Army attempted to employ DDT to control the spread of the disease, it had minimal success. Troops also suffered from exhaustion, malnutrition, and amoebic dysentery. Plane crashes and truck accidents occurred frequently across this difficult terrain.

Nurses stationed in isolated jungle hospitals in the Burma–India theater worked under primitive conditions in an extremely trying climate. Many served in the theater longer than the traditional two–year assignment and suffered from low morale. They performed a necessary task but often received little recognition in this demanding but forgotten theater of war.

Conclusion

In February 1945 U.S. troops liberated the sixty–seven Army nurses who had been imprisoned in Santo Tomas Internment Camp since 1942 and evacuated them to a convalescent hospital on Leyte. Although suffering from malnutrition and beriberi, they recovered from their ordeal fairly quickly. The duty they performed in combat and the hardships they endured as prisoners of war are testaments to the professionalism of the entire Army Nurse Corps throughout the war.

World War II ended with the surrender of Japan in September 1945, and Army nurses stationed around the world began planning to return home. They could look back on their service with great pride. Their accomplishments were many. Nurses had been a part of every link in the chain of evacuation established in every theater of the war. Their work contributed significantly to the low mortality rate experienced by American casualties of all types. Nurses received 1,619 medals, citations, and commendations during the war, reflecting the courage and dedication of all who served. Sixteen medals were awarded posthumously to nurses who died as a result of enemy fire. These included the 6 nurses who died at Anzio, 6 who died when the Hospital Ship *Comfort* was attacked by a Japanese suicide plane, and 4 flight nurses. Thirteen other flight nurses died in weather–related crashes while on duty. Overall, 201 nurses died while serving in the Army during the war.

Army nurses returning to civilian life discovered a changed postwar society. The place of women in American society had been irrevocably altered and expanded by the entrance of women into professional and industrial jobs previously reserved for men. Most important for nurses, however, was society's enhanced perception of nursing as a valued profession. The critical need for nurses and the federally funded Cadet Nurse Corps program had been well publicized during the war. Upon their return home, Army nurses were eligible for additional education under the G.I. Bill of Rights, which would enable them to pursue professional educational goals.

Veteran nurses also brought home with them valuable skills and experiences, increasing their professional status and self–esteem. The Army had trained significant numbers of nurses in specialties such as anesthesia and psychiatric care, and nurses who had served overseas had acquired practical experience otherwise unobtainable. Those assigned to field and evacuation hospitals had become accustomed to taking the initiative, making quick decisions, and adopting innovative solutions to a broad range of medical–related problems. They had learned organizational skills by moving and setting up field and evacuation hospitals while following the troops and had developed teaching and supervisory skills while training the corpsmen under their command. Paperwork no longer intimidated them, as circumstances had forced them to deal with increasingly complex administrative chores.

The Army nurse's experience forced her to grow professionally and gave her the self–confidence and opportunity to pursue her career when she returned to the United States. She came home to a society that was ready to accept nurses as professional members of the United States health care system. World War II had forever changed the face of military nursing.

Further Readings

There is no single comprehensive history of the U.S. Army Nurse Corps, nor is there a volume in the official United States Army in World War II series that deals with this corps. The best approach to learning more about Army nurses during World War II is to read the relatively few individual memoirs which have been published over the years. The following are among the best. In *From Nightingale to Eagle: An Army Nurses History* (1973), Edith A. Aynes describes her experiences as the chief nurse of the 148th General Hospital in Hawaii throughout 1942 and her eventual assignment to the Surgeon General's Office in Washington. Theresa Archard discusses her service with the 48th Surgical Hospital in North Africa in *GI Nightingale: The Story of an American Army Nurse* (1945). In *Jungle Angel: Bataan Remembered* (1988), Maxine K. Russell recounts the experiences of Army nurse Hortense E. McCay on Bataan.

Printed in the United Kingdom
by Lightning Source UK Ltd.
102613UKS00001B/84